W9-AIR-417

Disclaimer: This is a work of nonfiction and was written

for informational purposes only. You should not rely on

this information as a substitute for, nor does it replace,

professional medical advice, diagnosis, or treatment. If you have any concerns or questions about your or your child's health, you should always consult with a physician or other health-care professional. Do not disregard, avoid or delay obtaining medical or health related advice from your health-care professional because of something you may have read in this book. The use of any information provided in this book is solely at your own risk.

Contents

Introduction

Introduction: The Powerful Disease of Addiction

More people die from prescription drugs, heroin and now Fentanyl overdose than all the car crashes in the United States every year. It's not that the roads are better or cars and seat belts are safer, it's that the scourge of dangerous and illegal drugs has drastically spread throughout our country. This message came during a speech in West Virginia given by President Obama as he neared the end of his two terms as Commander in Chief of the United States.[1]

The disease of addiction is a physical and mental process that involves the reward centers of the brain, the rewarding stimulus (such as alcohol, tobacco or drugs) and the adverse behaviors and consequences that result. Guiding your child through the tumultuous years of adolescence to avoid substance abuse has never been more urgent and one of the many roles of parenting.[2]

I am an orthopaedic surgeon sub-specializing in spinal surgery with 30 years of experience in trauma centers from Miami to West Palm Beach and served in the United States Army Reserve Medical Corps as a surgeon stateside during the Gulf War. I have treated plenty of patients victimized by trauma or recovering from painful spinal surgery, many of whom required pain medication during the acute phase of recovery. Subsequently, some of those patients became addicted to the opioids used for their painful conditions.

My experience in helping patients cope with acutely painful conditions with safe, compassionate and quality medical care is standard practice; however, witnessing the downhill spiral of addiction for some is not unique. Any physician in the United States will have their own stories that relate to the powerful disease of addiction.

Many of my patients had injuries caused by trauma creating sufficient pain to need opioid painkillers like morphine, oxycodone and hydrocodone. Some may have already been addicted to alcohol, opioids or other substances prior to their trauma. It is humbling and instructive for a physician to witness the unintended consequences of treatment. Numerous people are affected with addiction that started by the appropriate prescribing and use of pain medicine. I have witnessed some of my own patients who never fully recovered from the disease of addiction face personal and private battles throughout their lifetime. No matter how it begins whether it is medically indicated with appropriate prescribed pain killers or a cascade of peer or social pressure, the disease of addiction, regardless of its origin, is one of the most tragic diseases.

As a surgeon, I am a fixer. When a bone is broken, I want to set it and watch it heal. When the skin is cut, I want to suture it up and watch it heal. But when a patient develops the disease of addiction, whether it is alcohol, drugs or tobacco, the fixer mentality in me is powerless. The pervasive nature of addiction does not lend itself to a quick fix.

As I reflect on the victims of trauma that I have treated over the years, from both military and civilian injuries, the importance of preventing and addressing the issue of addiction is reinforced. I have patients treated as teens and young adults that are older now, with families of their own that continue to fight the disease of addiction. I am also the father of six children, mostly all grown up, and three grandchildren. I share the concerns of all parents about the risks our children face as they grow up, but these concerns do not end once they are adults.

I applaud former President Obama for his willingness to address the problem of addiction head on and putting an honest effort to further federal resources into the management of this important and growing public health crisis in the United States. The 21st Century Cures Act, signed into law under his watch, allocated substantial resources to the battle against addiction. [3] The current President of the United States, Donald J. Trump, and his cabinet member, the Secretary of Health and Human Services, Dr. Tom Price, are in a strong position to continue this battle of historic proportions. Substance abuse and addiction in the United States is a crisis worthy of every possible effort.

The disease of addiction is powerful and does not discriminate based on race, gender or level of education. Tobacco, alcohol, opioids and other prescription and illicit drugs are chemically and behaviorally addictive substances that keep their victims in bondage. There are many basic scientific and clinical studies which explain the chemical and biological process of addiction. But all the science aside, the human toll of addiction to these substances is heartbreaking.

Addiction destroys passions, dreams and goals. It is a killer of innocence, opportunities and happiness. It is not overstated that each parent should do everything in their power to protect the quality of life of their child. Teaching good behavior by example, applying discipline from a position of love and concern, nurturing a child's ability to make good choices and to appreciate the consequences of poor choices is a parent's responsibility.

The purpose of this book is to provide insight into the reality of what our youth are facing and the tools to use as a guide to prepare them as they face it. Being a responsible parent is not easy for everyone. It does not depend on your geographical location or social and economic status. All parents are given the opportunity to bring up their children with love, support and understanding.

The following information has been collected from personal experience and published material. Parents are encouraged to research articles from government resources, rehabilitation centers and teen organizations to guide their children through the at-risk years. Collecting relevant information, gathering support from individuals who have been down this road and seeking advice from a professional therapist is essential in the fight against the disease of addiction. Prevention is far better than treatment. But once treatment is needed, facing the problem openly and compassionately and getting the help and support needed is critical.[4] Ultimately, it is up to each parent to take responsibility and turn awareness into action for the life of their child.

I. In a Perfect World

"I wish I could tell you it gets better but it doesn't get better. YOU get better." **Joan Rivers**[1]

Although this statement from Joan Rivers is referring to her life as a comedian, it is a clear representation of the challenges of parenting and life with kids.

In a perfect world, there would be no substance abuse or drug-related problems. In an ideal world, our kids would grow up as we expect them to with high moral standards living happy and successful lives. But, we live in a world that is far from perfect, and the choices our children make are not always under our control. In the real world, social pressures can cause compromises in behavior, shortcuts in actions, and at times, poor choices with consequences that can have devastating and lasting effects.

We live in a time where there is pressure on all fronts. Teens and young adults are especially under pressure to conform. They often feel it is important to act, dress and speak like their friends. I was raised in the '60's and '70's when bell bottoms and long hair was in, and I had both. My own children have grown up in the digital age with social media communications being the norm. Times change and it is important for parents to adapt.

The pressure placed on teens is unlike any other, and the reality is that at some point they will be faced with the presence of tobacco, drugs and alcohol. The choices they make at such a vulnerable and impressionable time can have a lasting impact on their quality of life and wellbeing.

No one chooses to be an addict. *Addiction is never the intent; it is however, often the end result of a choice made over and over that creates a physical and mental dependence.* Using or experimenting with addictive substances is the same as playing with fire, you eventually get burned. If you are experimenting with a substance, addiction will most likely be the outcome.

In the beginning, drugs, alcohol or tobacco may be used as an escape from anxiety or feelings of despondency or hopelessness, for pain relief from an injury or health condition, or in fun and to fit in with the crowd. Tobacco products, alcoholic beverages and many drugs are highly addictive substances and over time form a habit, then dependence and ultimately a physical and mental addiction.[2]

There is no genetic makeup or strength of character that prevents the human body from becoming addicted. Many substances with potential for abuse are widely available and often inexpensive. Whether obtained from a friend, purchased on the street or prescribed by a well-meaning physician, substances can be abused. Abuse can lead to addiction and tragic consequences.

In my practice, some patients including teens and young adults that seek treatment for neck or back pain are often already dependent on tobacco products, alcohol, pain killers or other substances. As a spine surgeon, the treatment of addiction is outside my specialty, so I refer such patients to other doctors that have experience in managing addictions. Pain management specialists, psychologists, psychiatrists, and many internal and family medicine practitioners are experienced in helping manage the health consequences of addiction.

We all face personal struggles – it's a part of life that comes with the journey. No one gets a free ride. Having teens amuse themselves or succumb to peer pressure and experiment with alcohol or drugs may seem like minor reckless and even common behavior but most recovering addicts will tell you they started using between the ages of 12 and 17.[3]

The disease of addiction has created a large population of Americans that need professional help. It is particularly sad to see the vitality and opportunity of youth dampened by addiction. I have known many people from patients to friends, family members and colleagues that have become addicted to one or another substance over their lifetime. I do not know even one that would say that cigarettes, alcohol or drugs were ever worth it. Most would say if they could turn back the clock, they would not have taken that first hit, drink, pill or injection.

The tragic part is that those who never fully recover from their addiction miss out on many of life's joys and opportunities. Alternatively, individuals in recovery or even those who stopped experimenting early on, generally lead normal, productive and enjoyable lives.

II. Driving Under the Influence

"My teenage years were exactly what they were supposed to be. Everybody has their own path. It's laid out for you. It's just up to you to walk it."
Justin Timberlake[1]

Even though loaning your car to your teenager can cause some anxiety, many teens are responsible drivers. However, others may not have matured enough to be safe, responsible and considerate behind the wheel. Auto insurance companies charge a larger premium for drivers under the age of 25 due to the higher risk of texting, driving while under the influence or just being reckless. The Centers for Disease Control and Prevention (CDC) report that accidents are the leading cause of death for teens ages 15-19 in the United States and car fatalities are at the top of that category.[2] It is crucial during the teenage years to instill responsibility and accountability for all actions, and driving is one of them.

According to the CDC, excessive drinking in the United States has reached $249 billion in health care costs with $171 billion from binge drinking. Binge drinking is defined as four or more alcoholic beverages for each occurrence.[3] The statistics from the National Institute on Alcohol Abuse and Alcoholism (NIAAA) reveal that youth in the U.S. have now started drinking at a younger age than ever before. Similar numbers of boys and girls engage in binge drinking. However, teenage boys tend to binge drink more than teenage girls.[4]

There are significant dangers related to those drinking under the age of 21, and it's important to understand the risks and consequences. The NIAAA reported on data collected from the CDC that underage drinking has been a factor in an estimated 4,358 deaths each year from 2006-2010. These fatalities included automobile accidents, homicides, alcohol poisoning, falls, drowning, and suicides. In 2015, teen fatalities involving auto accidents remained significantly high. The NIAAA also states that 11% of the alcohol intake in the U.S. is consumed by young people ages 12 to 20. Alcohol is abused more commonly by teens than any illegal drug.[5] The lost opportunities and tragic consequences for surviving family and friends are incomprehensible.

As a father of six and a team physician for a local high school for over fifteen years, I have witnessed countless numbers of youth devastated by alcohol and drug-related trauma. There will always be tragic accidents, but it is the increase in the number of deaths every year from potent and readily available substances that must be addressed. While every accident cannot be eliminated, it is everyone's responsibility to bring awareness of this subject to the teen community. Collective actions by motivated adult citizens will ultimately save lives.

In addition to car accidents, underage drinking causes impaired judgment leading to risky sexual activity and behavioral problems. It places teens in danger of becoming victims of sexual or physical assault. Alcohol not only impairs judgment, it also interferes with brain function and structure. The human brain continues to develop well into the twenties and alcohol is a poison that adversely effects brain development. *Childhood and teenage years are crucial stages for development and substances have the power to alter normal healthy brain maturation.*[6]

Even subtle damage to the developing adolescent brain from underage or binge drinking may cause cognitive problems, such as loss of focus, problem solving difficulty, and degraded academic skills. Alcohol addiction can start in the teen years and continue for a lifetime. Alcohol intoxication causes a change in emotional states, such as mood, lowered physical capabilities, fuzzy thinking, blurred vision, speech impairment, bizarre behavior, poor judgment and loss of interest in appearance.[7]

There are many reasons teenagers or young adults feel the need or desire to drink. One often stated reason is to relax and have fun. When teens drink, they feel less stress.[8] But by decreasing the emotional and physical self-preservation behaviors called inhibitions, alcohol may increase confidence and create a false sense of courage. Realistically, alcohol is an intoxicating and addictive depressant that only worsens the existing social or emotional pressures that teens experience.[9] Teenage years can be tough on everyone, so it's important to remember the level of pressure and expectations placed on teens and young adults. In my experience where children are concerned, nothing good comes from alcohol, drug or tobacco use.

As a parent, teacher or coach, there are many things that can be done to counteract the harmful effects and dangerous behaviors that are directly related to underage drinking. We can begin by openly communicating the consequences of abusing alcohol. Make no mistake, underage drinking is alcohol abuse. Underage drinking and driving under the influence has led to tragic consequences that most of us would not want to suffer.
I offer seven ways to communicate changes and conversations into your home, school or team that will help nurture positive and healthy relationships.[10]

1. Lead by example. Parents, coaches and teachers, if you choose to drink, do so responsibly. Don't drink and drive and don't drink to excess. Be an effective role model. Children are observing everything you do.
2. Discuss the risks, dangers and consequences of consuming alcohol. Open communication is necessary to get

the message across. As a physician, I can tell you that teenagers and most others are unaware that brain tissue and neuronal connections continue to develop from childhood into the twenties. Drinking alcohol in these formative years may play a part in complicating that development.

3. Do not encourage or enable underage or binge drinking. However, if they choose to do so, speak about the responsibilities and repercussions that are appropriate for your family.

4. Do not make alcohol easily available in your home. Keeping alcohol or substances out of your home lessens the chance of it becoming a source.

5. Communicate openly and frequently with parents involved in your child's life. Sleepovers, parties, vacations and road trips are many times an invitation to underage and binge drinking. Set the standards and limitations and share your style of discipline with the other parents.

Communicate what is and what is not appropriate.

6. Offer to supervise parties and events or communicate with someone that does. Make a firm and well thought out decision on whether or not your teen should attend the party. While it is important to respectfully consider your teen's requests, it is ultimately your decision.

7. Listen to your child without judgment. Empathy is necessary for compassion. While it is not possible to walk in their shoes or share in all of their experiences, looking at your child's life from that perspective will improve social connectedness. It doesn't mean that you should give in to the demands of your teenager, but understanding why they have those demands helps. Strive to gain knowledge about your child's life outside of the home without too much intrusiveness. Doing so will provide insight and clues about what's going on in their lives.

It may not be easy to speak with your child or any youth about difficult and sensitive subjects, but in my experience, it is extremely important to maintain lines of communication and let them know the boundaries and consequences.[11] If you suspect or are aware that your child is abusing alcohol or any substance, it is imperative to get help. Understand what you're dealing with and do the research. Resources for support include counselors, family therapists, and treatment programs.

As a parent, if you become aware of any rebellious or unacceptable behavior, the task of confronting your child can be daunting, but take heart, you are not the first, nor will you be the last parent to do so. The first step is to sit down with your child and have an open and honest conversation. While it may be a difficult conversation, it is necessary to explain that behaviors have consequences. Showing compassion will enable the one you're talking with to feel safe and connected. It takes emotional effort to confront a teenager, even your own, but it will be worth it in the long run to turn anyone away from a life of addiction, even if they don't realize it or appreciate it.

III.   The Upside to Adversity

"The journey of a thousand miles begins with a single step." **Lao Tzu**[1]

Many parents make it a point to keep their child from dealing with the hardships of life. While there is a range of parenting behaviors, it is innate for a parent to protect their child. It's what we all do in some form or fashion. However, in my opinion, allowing youth to face their own struggles and work through them can enable a sense of responsibility. **Adversity can become a catalyst in building strength and character.** Each parent must set their own boundaries and implement them with love and compassion.

Overcoming adversity has been a common thread among those who have achieved great things and attained success.[2] Looking back at history or peering into the lives and thoughts of current accomplished individuals has merit. Here are a few examples of achieving success over adversity.

❖ **Franklin D. Roosevelt** served our country as President of the United

States four terms and saw the country through the Great Depression and World War II. At 39 years old, he was paralyzed from the waist down by polio.[3]

- ❖ **LeBron James**, professional basketball player for the NBA, winning three national titles stated the biggest obstacles he overcame was going through the struggles he went through as a kid and not taking it personal. "Going through obstacles and hopping over speed bumps and the trials and tribulations I went through as a kid helped me get here [NBA]".[4]

- ❖ **Oprah Winfrey**, multi-award winning talk show host, producer, actress and one of the greatest philanthropists in this era suffered significant hardships during her childhood. She states "she became an excellent student after a turning point in her life when she went to live with her father who provided structure, guidance rules and books."[2,5]

- ❖ **Dr. Paul Edward Farmer**, Harvard-trained physician and medical anthropologist, and Kolokotrones University Professor of Global Health and Social Medicine. He is a champion of health and human rights for the poorest of poor in the impoverished island country of Haiti. Professor Farmer is the founding director of Partners in Health an International Non-profit Organization. I became familiar with PIH from my own medical work in Haiti. He grew up in a working class but very poor family. Through dedication to education, a limitless work-ethic, and profound compassion for those most in need, Dr. Farmer has become a role model for countless physicians across the world. He is mine. He defines the concept of altruism that many health-care and humanitarian aid workers aspire to in their career.

Allowing your child to face adversity and disappointments while **guiding them to use proper channels will teach them coping skills, emotional resilience, creative thinking and**

the ability to collaborate. Children going into their middle and high school years can enter this phase with confidence, focus, creativity and expressiveness by giving them the tools they need for independence and the encouragement to use them. [6] Our five adult children have developed uniqueness as individuals with favorable character traits: a teacher, a U.S. Marine, a musician, a physical therapist, and a police officer in training, while the sixth is still in high school preparing to pursue her goals and dreams.

Staying alert and aware of your child's environment, the friends they hang with, who they are attracted to and allowing them to solve problems with guidance, love and emotional support will serve them well in the end.

IV. The Pressure is On

"Everything negative – pressure, challenges – is all an opportunity for me to rise."
Kobe Bryant[1]

If it hasn't happened already, you can be sure that at some point your teen will be pressured to drink alcohol, smoke marijuana, take pain medication or 'hook-up' with many other drug-related scenarios. If you suspect that your child might be experimenting with drugs or alcohol, you may be right. As a parent, it is easy to be unprepared for this phase of your child's life. Friends and acquaintances often have a stronger influence on a teen's behavior than the parent.[2]

Be comforted by the fact that it's completely natural for teens to experiment and learn things on their own; it's how they learn to be an adult and find their own identity. At this phase, it is best to be supportive and create an open environment for communication to stay connected with your child. It is always the parent's responsibility to be aware of their children's environment and what's going on in the community. The drug crisis is no longer an inner city problem; it has permeated into the urban and rural areas of the country and in the current era of ultra-potent synthetic drugs, one pill may be their last.

If your child is consistently defying the rules and expectations you've established, showing tough love works for some during this phase, but it may alienate your child, which would be counterproductive to the intent. However, being a push-over parent and accepting behaviors and choices that are destructive and damaging can setup your child for a lifetime of failure.[3] Making consistent unrestrained poor choices contribute to lost opportunities and dire consequences.

Tough love can be a compassionate alternative if your child shows no interest in compromising, negotiating or modifying his behavior. Other family members are made to suffer when there's rebellion in the family. Demonstrating tough love in our household is taking a firm stand that allows the child to experience the consequences of his actions, but not to the extreme. Tough love does not involve abuse or neglect, nor is it giving up on the individual regardless of poor choices and questionable behaviors.[4] Each family has its own boundaries and style of discipline. Take ownership of yours and be consistent, your child will benefit from that stability.[5]

Reaching out to connect with your teen by listening with undivided attention, giving liberty in decision making on appearance, hobbies and sports and acknowledging strengths may deliver greater results. Discipline and consequences are important, but what is most important is the relationship with your child.[6] Parents with a teen who is using drugs or alcohol should enlist the help of a family therapist specifically trained in substance abuse.

Educating yourself on the current trend of drugs and taking the steps to build a foundation of trust, discipline, compassion and love may help to avoid the initial problems of addiction and enable your family to triumph over the odds.

V.   Statistically Speaking

"Education is the most powerful weapon which you can use to change the world."
Nelson Mandela[1]

As mentioned in the introduction, it is reported by the CDC that more people now die in the United States from prescription drug and heroin overdose than the number from car crashes. Moreover, prescription drugs claim more lives every year than heroin and cocaine combined.[2] I expect this trend to change as physicians tighten their prescribing practices while chemists and drug dealers further invade the United States with cheap, powerful and dangerous synthetic drugs. In my observation, there is no doubt that synthetic opioids and designer drugs are gaining a foothold in the U.S.

Physicians are ever more aware of the dangers posed by prescribing opioids. The medical profession is proactive at optimizing the quality, safety and compassion in medical care which includes prescribing pain medication. Despite efforts to fight this epidemic, death from drug overdoses especially opioids remain unacceptably high.

In my view, synthetic opioids of the Fentanyl and Carfentanil class, and illegal synthetics with hallucinogenic and stimulant properties pose a clear and present danger to health and wellbeing in the United States.[3] They are linked to a spike in the overdose death rate due to the increased potency and the associated respiratory depression. A lethal overdose, even a small amount of substance, can kill the victim in minutes. When the brain is not triggering the biologic drive to breathe, lack of oxygenated blood to organs quickly causes death by cardiac arrest. Synthetic opioids are considerably more potent, and often less expensive than morphine or heroin. Dealers have been known to lace the heroin supply with synthetics to increase strength while lowering cost. The dealers are now lacing pills and using pill stamping machines to give the appearance of prescription legitimacy to counterfeit opioids.[4]

The benzodiazepines, such as Xanax and Valium, are also highly addictive medications reasonably prescribed by doctors to treat anxiety, muscle spasms and other clinical problems. These medications have also become one of the many common prescription drugs middle and high school students are abusing.[5] Opioid addiction will create weeks of painful withdrawal symptoms following discontinued use of medication without a substitute, but it is rarely life threatening. The same is not true for benzodiazepine withdrawal; the chemical reactions of these drugs on the brain can lead to fatal consequences. The National Institute on Drug Abuse reported that since 2010, heroin and synthetic opioids have propelled an increase in cocaine-related overdose deaths, even though the popularity of cocaine has been on the decline. These new findings are consistent with the increasing trend of opioid, heroin and illegally sold fentanyl.[6]

Prescription drug abuse is defined as someone using medication that was not prescribed for them or taking prescribed medicine for reasons other than advised, according to the Mayo Clinic. Inadvertent or incorrect use of a prescribed drug is not considered abuse. The overuse and abuse of prescription pain medicines and anti-anxiety medications has reached rampant proportions, and has become a nationwide health crisis.[7]

As a surgeon treating acute spinal pain and post-surgical pain, I am aware that prescription medications may be misused, abused and illegally sold for profit. Sometimes patients confuse medications. Many times patients don't realize medication can interact with other drugs, alcohol or even food causing adverse reactions. The prescribing physician, a pharmacist and even a credible website can all be valid sources for information about medication. Prescribed medications may also be diverted from the intended patient to someone else. Even if you think you're helping out a friend or family, this is ill advised and illegal.[8] When prescription drugs especially those categorized as "controlled substances," by the Drug Enforcement Agency (DEA) are misdirected from the intended patient to someone else, legal consequences can follow. The DEA takes the management of controlled substances seriously. The only legal and advised way to access prescription drugs is to have a doctor's prescription.[9]

A healthy community is founded on commitment to the wellbeing of its families. The family unit, friends and neighbors create a sense of cohesiveness and strength for support and sustainability. It takes a community of people to stand and work together to battle

e crisis of substance abuse. **When your child**
, abusing substances of any kind, awareness
s the first step to any resolution. Parents must
be willing to acknowledge the condition
affecting their child and have an open
conversation, especially with an expert.
Connecting with a therapist trained in substance
abuse can help to identify and address the
underlying issues behind the use of drugs and
alcohol. Counseling, therapy and rehabilitation
will go a long way in helping with abstinence
and recovery.

It's common parental behavior to ignore the
signs of substance abuse or addiction and hope
the problem will just go away. But denial only
worsens a situation, while acceptance allows
you to work toward a solution. Facing the
problem head on and seeking help can often
prevent escalation from alcohol or drug
abuse. As a father, I know firsthand the
tendency of a parent to want to avoid an issue.
Confrontation is uncomfortable. If you become
aware that your child may be experimenting
with or using drugs or alcohol, it is important to
take the proper steps and to do so quickly.
Getting accurate information about the type and
amount of substance your child is using and

taking appropriate action will empower you and your family to make positive changes. Your child does not have to become another statistic. You have the ability right now to change the course of your child's future by taking the appropriate action and getting the right help and support.

VI.   Drug of Choice

The drug of choice is a term commonly used to note the preference of one drug over another, as an addict or as a treating physician. [1] Natural opioid drugs come from natural opium alkaloids, derived from the poppy plant. Opioids have a physiologic effect of relieving pain and while there are quite a few natural opioids, the most common include: morphine, codeine and heroin. [2]

Overdoses of prescription drugs and heroin continue to be the leading cause of unintentional death for Americans rising 14 percent from 2013 to 2014.[3] The CDC also reports the death rates from synthetic opioids have increased 72.2 percent from 2014 to 2015. Synthetic opioids are considered painkillers manufactured in labs with a similar chemical structure to a natural opiate drug. Synthetic opioids can be medications that are legally prescribed by doctors or illicit drugs found on the streets with small molecular differences that create unreliable potency. Some examples of synthetic opioids are Fentanyl, Methadone and Meperidine, also known as Demerol.[4]

Semi-synthetic opioids are potent painkillers that can be dangerous and come at a great risk for abuse. Some common semi-synthetics widely in use by healthcare providers are hydrocodone or oxycodone. If the substance has naturally been taken from the poppy plant and then chemically altered in the manufacturing process it is considered semi-synthetic. Either way, opioids natural, synthetic or semi-synthetic have the potential for abuse and addiction. Opioids should only be taken under the direction of a physician. These drugs come with a high risk of physical, mental and emotional dependency, detachment and addiction.[5]

It is widely known that drugs can have dangerous effects. Prescription pain killers are high-risk because they are prescribed as the first line of treatment for pain, easily accessible and highly addictive. Everyone experiences pain at some level, at some time in life. A common solution for fast and easy relief is to take prescription pain medicine.

Most teens believe that prescription drugs are safer than illegal street drugs. A recent survey conducted by drugfreeworld.org reveals *70 percent of teens that abuse these drugs stated that home medicine cabinets were their source.* [6] Pain medicine can be used appropriately and under the supervision of a physician for temporary as well as chronic pain. Pain medicine can also be a danger depending on where and how it is stored. I recommend to my patients that it should be locked up and discarded when the use for the pain medicine has passed. Do not store pain medicine in case you need it in the future. It is always best to return unused pain medication to the pharmacy for safe disposal.

Although measures have been taken to address the epidemic of substance abuse and addiction, the numbers of non-fatal and fatal overdose continue to escalate. The CDC reported the fatality rate from prescription opioids including oxycodone and hydrocodone has quadrupled since 1999.[7] Recreational drugs in the form of illegally misdirected pain pills remain far too available. Even as relatively inexpensive, Fentanyl-laced heroin and Fentanyl-laced counterfeit pain pills sweep the country, creating an ongoing threat to both addicts and those experimenting recreationally. This threat should keep parents awake at night and creates a call-to-action that must not be ignored. While there is not one simple solution, prevention and early intervention can save lives, create opportunities for well-being and circumvent the disease of addiction.

The principles and logic of harm reduction in the battle against addiction has great merit. The concepts, policies and practices address measures to lower the risk of disease, social isolation and death from the use of psychoactive drugs that the user is unable to stop. Harm reduction lowers the spread of HIV and hepatitis through simple and inexpensive needle-exchange programs. The risk of death by overdose is lowered by safe zones in which the respiratory depression of accidental overdose can be mitigated. As a physician, I find the concepts of harm reduction compassionate and appropriate for a society such as the United States, and others. However, the stigma of disease of addiction carries social and political baggage that limits the widespread implementation of harm reduction practices.

The most popular synthetic drugs are synthetic marijuana and "bath salts". Use of these synthetic drugs can lead to a temporary high or permanent hallucinogenic state with long lasting psychotic/nervous system effects. Cognitive changes from ingesting these drugs can create harmful effects to the nervous system. Even recreational use of a synthetic drug carries an extreme health threat with a high risk of overdose and possibility of death.[8] The antidote drug for an opioid overdose, Narcan, is a prescription medicine that comes in a nasal spray and is available in many states. If the user becomes unresponsive, it must be administered immediately, but it is not a substitute for emergency medical care, nor is it a cure for addiction.[9]

There are many synthetic drugs that exist on the street. They are known as LSD, Meth (methamphetamine), Ecstasy (MDMA), Rohypnol, PCP, OxyContin, and surprisingly the most accessible and popular are bath salts. Synthetic drugs are also found in the form of pharmaceuticals, and some are available in local markets and head shops. There exists a race between state and federal authorities identifying and classifying the newly emerging synthetic drugs while chemists are actively working in labs creating new formulas. In my opinion, the disease of addiction requires law enforcement involvement as well as community measures of prevention, rehabilitation and recovery.[10]

Cannabinoids are a group of active compounds found in the Cannabis plant, also referred to as marijuana. The two compounds that are the most prominent are THC, tetrahydrocannabinol, a mind-altering ingredient, and CBD, a non-psychoactive cannabinoid.[11]

The National Institute on Drug Abuse, (NIDA), reports that THC causes psychological effects similar to the chemicals made naturally by the body by attaching to the receptors in the brain associated with thoughts, memory, time perception, pleasure and coordination. The NIDA also reports THC has been known to induce "delusions, hallucinations and, in some cases anxiety, elation, sedation, short-term memory loss and pain relief."[12]

Synthetic drugs are considered designer drugs when chemically altered to avoid having it classified as illegal. Just a slight modification of a chemical side-chain can circumvent the DEA. What began as an experiment by a chemist, with the intention of creating a new drug that could be sold legally on the internet or in stores, has turned into an entire criminal enterprise. The goal is for dealers to make money without breaking the law. Some of these drugs are sold over the internet as herbal smoking blends.[13]

These drugs, also known as "new psychoactive substances" imitate the mind-altering effects of illegal drugs and were banned for only serving the purpose of getting high without any other medical benefit. Some of the names of these cannabinoids are "K2, Blaze, Genie, Red X Dawn, Spice and Zohai." These substances can be smoked, made into tea or purchased as liquid to smoke in a vaporizer. The common side effects of these drugs are "nausea, vomiting, rapid heart rate, severe agitation, anxiety, elevated blood pressure, tremors, seizures, hallucinations, dilated pupils, violent behavior and suicidal thoughts."[14]

There is a new powerful drug on the street, and it goes by the name of "Flakka", often referred to as the "zombie" drug. Flakka is a synthetic cathinone, more commonly known as bath salts. Synthetic cathinone substances can be much stronger than the natural product and very dangerous. The drug comes in the form of white or pink crystals resembling rock candy or fish tank "gravel", another common name. This drug is highly addictive with stimulant effects. It increases heart rate, energy and alertness. [15] But the heightened adrenaline effect comes at a grave price to the mind and body of the user.

Individuals consume Flakka by injecting, snorting or putting it into vapes or e-cigarettes. The body may react to Flakka by going into hyperthermia, increasing the body temperature higher than 105 degrees, which in turn causes "extreme paranoia and agitation, hallucinations, and super human strength." An adrenaline surge feeds the paranoia, creating the illusion that the user is being followed or chased. The police department of Broward County in Florida reports that it will sometimes require four to five police officers to restrain or capture an individual who is using Flakka because of excessive strength and adrenaline.[16]

Other dangers and complications of using Flakka include excited "delirium, seizures and metabolic problems" due to muscle over-activity, dehydration and rhabdomyolysis, a process where muscle tissue breaks down releasing proteins and other cellular products he bloodstream, clogging and poisoning dneys. The result of dehydration and omyolysis can lead to renal failure or death.[17] A lifetime of kidney dialysis or a kidney transplant for those that survive should be frightening enough for the young substance abuser to avoid bath salts. Without this knowledge, teens may be oblivious. It is every parent's, family member's, coach's or teacher's responsibility to educate those under their supervision on the dangers of bath salts, other drugs, alcohol and tobacco. While alcohol and tobacco may seem less harmful in comparison, drinking to excess and smoking will lead to significant problems of their own.

My father was Chief of Police of Greenacres, Florida when I was growing up in the 1970's. Even though Flakka was non-existent at that time, there were plenty of marijuana, alcohol and drunk-driving scenarios that kept my father busy. Having my father serve as the Chief of Police in my small southern town helped keep me on the straight and narrow. Getting accepted to Columbia University for college, and then the University of Miami for medical school had much to do with a strong and positive parental influence. All parents are given the opportunity to be a positive influence and role model in their child's life. Mine certainly were and I aspire to that with my children.

VII. The Drug Enforcement Agency

The Drug Enforcement Agency (DEA) had no reported cases involving Flakka in 2010; however, that number escalated to 670 in 2014. The journal *Psychopharmacology* showed findings that Flakka was more addictive than methamphetamine.[1]

In 2014, the DEA reported that Broward County, Florida, led the nation in Flakka cases. The drug, chemically known as alpha-PVP, was manufactured in clandestine labs in China.[2] Availability is made easily through local street-drug markets and online mail-order businesses. This drug is also more accessible and affordable than many other drugs. The DEA has been credited for the ban of 115 chemical substances and synthetic drugs resulting in lowered cases of Flakka and synthetic cannabinoids. DEA officials are optimistic that meetings with Chinese counterparts will help solve the synthetic drug crisis in the United States. As mentioned, the problem that the DEA in the United States and drug agencies in

China are now facing is keeping up with the chemists that are changing formulas to stay ahead of the laws.[3]

DEA spokesman Russell Baer says, "Historically, we have not been able to talk about this stuff [with Chinese counterparts]. We've now gotten to the point that China is listening to us and addressing some of the [drug] scheduling issues. They are their own country, and they have their own concerns. One [problem] people don't understand is that China has an extensive commercial manufacturing program over there. These illicit substances ... are a small part of that huge legitimate industry." While the DEA has recently reported a decline in cases involving Flakka, there is still concern of trafficking and distribution.[4]

In 2016, the DEA added five synthetic opioids to the list of banned substances that have no medical purpose and pose a significant risk of abuse. Fentanyl-related drugs are powerful opioids similar to morphine, but 50 to 100 times more potent. Fentanyl is a prescription drug used to treat patients that suffer severe pain, cancer pain or to help manage pain during and after surgery. Anesthesiologists have long used these and other opioids to ease patients safely through surgery. The prescription names for Fentanyl are Actiq®, Duragesic®, and Sublimaze®. When drugs like heroin are laced with Fentanyl and sold on the streets, they are referred to as "China Girl, China White, Apache, Dance Fever, Goodfella, Jackpot, Murder 8, TNT, and Tango and Cash." [5]

There are increasing reports of the drug, Fentanyl, being added as a cocktail to substances such as morphine and other common prescription pain pills. It is not a coincidence that opioids are popular drugs for abuse. The effects of these drugs produce a state of euphoria, which is a mental state of extreme pleasure, excitement and well-being. Opioids affect the user by raising the level of dopamine in the brain. This medicinal effect tends to control pain and alter emotions. The negative medical side effects of opioids involve "confusion, nausea, drowsiness, sedation, addiction, respiratory depression, unconsciousness, coma and death." [6]

Lysergic acid diethylamide, better known as LSD or acid is a psychedelic drug known for its psychological effects. Hallucinogens, such as LSD and Ecstasy, are popular among pre-teens and teenagers today. LSD is derived from lysergic acid, which is found in a fungus that grows on rye and other grains. Another synthetic hallucinogen kids are using goes by the innocuous name Special K, or Ketamine. Ketamine is used as an anesthetic by veterinarians and physicians. These are powerful and lethal drugs that are sold on the streets as well.[7]

MDMA (methylenedioxy-methamphetamine), also known as Ecstasy or Molly, is another popular substance in the nightclub scene and high school parties. Chemically, this drug is a mixture of stimulants and hallucinogens that gives the user an effect of high energy, emotions of pleasure, distorted sensory and time perception. Most users purchase this drug in hope of a "pure" crystalline powder form of MDMA, typically sold in capsule form. However, many times users are deceitfully sold bath salts. This is another major risk of buying any drug on the street.[8]

VIII. Casual Conversation

Being a teenager today is harder than ever. And while not all teens are rebellious, the stress of deadlines for homework, reports and projects, the nervous tension of a test, the demanding pressure to conform, plus the evolution of social media combine to create a superficial sense of identity and anxiety.

In 2013, the Partnership Attitude Tracking Study (PATS) estimated that 20 percent of kids that learn about the risks of drugs from their parents are less likely to use drugs, while 20 percent of kids that used drugs reported not getting that benefit.[1]

As a parent, in order to have an understanding of this urgency and stress, it is crucial to build rapport with your teen by having conversations that provide comfort, trust and security. Don't wait until your child is heading off to college.[2] Starting with casual conversations when your child is younger is important. The simple act of reading to young children every day provides an opportunity to communicate in a non-confrontational manner. There are a number of books for children available that teach principles and character. This is a great method for building a warm and lasting relationship and guiding young children into their impressionable and formative years.

The NIDA reveals that "25 percent of those who started abusing prescription drugs at age 13 or younger develop a substance use disorder at some point in their life...". Statistics from the AddictionCenter.com tells us that more than 20 million individuals 12 years of age and over are in current need of treatment for substance abuse and addiction; ages 18 to 25 have the highest rate for illegal drug use; most of those with an addiction started smoking, drinking or using illegal drugs before the age of 18.[3,4]

While these findings are terrifying, they are informative and realistic. Don't avoid conversations out of denial or by assuming that your child will "just say no" to drugs and alcohol. **We live in an ever-changing world with many dangers and pressures on our youth. The role of a parent is to stay aware to protect, support and nurture them.** Parents are the ones that can make a difference in the lives of children. The hope is to prevent future problems.[5]

As mentioned, an inadvertent overdose of Fentanyl, mixed into a pain pill, can cause death from respiratory depression in 5 to10 minutes. While not every pre-teen or teenager will experiment with drugs, it is an unrealistic expectation to believe that it will never happen to yours. Drug experimentation, abuse and addiction do not discriminate; drug abuse resides in schools, down the street and maybe in your house. Addiction destroys relationships, families and lives. No one wants their child to become addicted to drugs, alcohol or even tobacco. Our lives are a gift to be lived with purpose, but finding our purpose is not always easy. What matters is that your child finds purpose and learns how to deal with stress, anxiety, disappointments, unexpected outcomes and tragedies.

IX. Suspect Behavior: When All Signs Point to Drug Use

"And I'll find strength in pain, and I will change my ways, I'll know my name as it's called again..."
The Cave, Mumford and Sons[1]

There are *specific signs and behavioral changes* that are displayed when someone is abusing substances. Drug users have common behavior traits that include the tendency to lie more often, manipulate others or continually shift blame. Students may lose interest in academics and extra-curricular activities and grades may begin to drop. Excitability or depression may become prominent and their desire and motivation to achieve may lessen over time.[2]

As a parent, you may notice a difference in your teen's personality and behaviors, although it is common to overlook such changes. They may develop slowly over time making substance abuse difficult to recognize.

When it comes to physical symptoms, the user may have "bloodshot or glazed eyes, dilated or constricted pupils, abrupt weight changes, bruises, infections" or other physical signs. If the user begins to have a runny nose consistently along with other symptoms, she may be snorting some type of substance. If the user is wearing long sleeves more often when short sleeves are more appropriate, he may be injecting substances.[3]

Behavioral changes that may appear when someone is using drugs include "increased aggression, irritability, lethargy, depression, anxiety, sudden changes in socializing, financial problems that cannot be explained, sleep changes, excessive sweating, paranoia, memory loss, and even criminal activity." These are the common behavioral changes to watch for if you suspect substance abuse.[4]

Being proactive and paying close attention to any situation regarding your teen may provide insight to what is going on. Once you have the facts, taking appropriate action with professional support is essential. It is important to be vigilant, **but nothing alienates a child more quickly than a parent who jumps to conclusions.**

As a surgeon, I manage many patients who have severe acute pain from trauma and surgery, including teens and young adults. It has been reported that doctors in my field, orthopaedic surgery for management of musculoskeletal trauma and diseases, are responsible for around seven percent of all opioid prescriptions in the United States. In my experience, some of the signs and symptoms of drug abuse can easily masquerade as typical teenage adolescent behavior.

X.   The Life of Addiction

"My identity shifted when I got into recovery. That's who I am now, and it actually gives me greater pleasure to have that identity than to be a musician or anything else, because it keeps me in a manageable size." **Eric Clapton**[1]

"Using" is the slang word to describe the illicit or illegal use of drugs. Most users experience drastic changes in their life the more often they use. They may experience loss of control, the inability to stop using, neglecting other activities that used to be important and less socializing with family or friends.[2]

When users reach the point of addiction, their tolerance increases and the need for any type of high intensifies. If they are unable to get the physical high, they may experience withdrawal symptoms, such as "anxiety, trembling, sweating, nausea, vomiting, pain, insomnia, severe depression, irritability, fatigue, loss of appetite, and headaches." At this point, the user needs medical attention and support. She has reached the point of addiction and may not be able to stop using or have the desire to quit. The user may now be experiencing all types of powerful emotions and problems as the focus is on feeding the addiction and finding the next high.[3]

When trying to help an addict, your attempts may seem futile. The user is completely disconnected and unable to exhibit gratitude or acknowledge your effort and desire to help him. **At this level of addiction, it is imperative to enlist the help of an expert and find a supportive network.** At some point, a professional therapist with specialized training in substance abuse may recommend taking legal action such as imposing the Baker Act or Marchman Act. Don't let fear dissuade you from helping your child.[4]

In 2016, the federal government passed guidelines to give physicians direction in their prescribing methods for opioids and benzodiazepines. It is encouraging to see medical society, federal and state governments and individual physicians take steps to stem the flow of painkillers. Although there are many recognized and legitimate medical reasons to prescribe pain killers, meticulous attention to the ethical guidelines in the practice of medicine, especially in the prescribing of controlled substances (regulated by the DEA) is critical.

XI. When You're Teen is Out of Control

When it comes to illicit drugs, marijuana is the most commonly used. However, with the expanding number of states that have loosened the laws regarding the use of marijuana products, opinions and recommendations about the drug are debatable and under transformation.

Other drugs teens are using to get high include: amphetamines, Adderall, opioid painkillers, Cannibinoids, tranquilizers, cough medicine, hallucinogens, sedatives, LSD, Ecstasy, Cocaine, Ritalin, Vicodin, OxyContin and inhalants.[1] Every year, there are reported deaths for nearly every drug listed. Currently, the average age of heroin addicts in treatment is 23. When surveyed, high school students reported being able to access drugs through friends, word of mouth, a parent's prescriptions and the internet. When asked which drugs were being sold, the answers were marijuana, prescription drugs, cocaine and ecstasy.[2,3]

Even in the 1970's, my father, dealt with teens "huffing" and inhaling all types of volatile chemicals including ether used for car engines. History has a way of repeating itself. As a physician, I am a strong proponent of treatment programs and advise patients to appropriately dispose of their prescription drugs, especially pain killers, once the clinical condition and need for the medication has passed. Pharmacies are prepared to manage this disposal by accepting the bottle of medication so that there will be no risk for misuse and misdirection at home. In addition, storing any type of pain killers in your cabinet is an invitation for others to misappropriate and abuse prescription drugs.

While we are not able to control every decision our child or teenager makes, as parents we can practice some preventative measures in the hope of avoiding the path of addiction. Once a child reaches junior high school age 11-13 there will begin a transition period. He may begin to question authority and parents' views on issues and start listening more to peers. This critical age requires additional effort on the parental side and sensitivity to these changes.[4] Once your child has reached 13-15 years of age, they may have been exposed to tobacco, drugs and alcohol or even experimented with it. Early high school years require extra vigilance on your part by creating open communication and setting ground rules with consequences.[5]

Make a real effort to pay attention and notice what your child is interested in and discuss it daily. Remember to give positive affirmation as well when your child is being honest and working hard. These years are an extremely difficult time for your child. Adolescents are searching for a sense of identity to relate to their friends, social media and adults. For high school students who are 16-18 years of age, the opportunities to make time for conversation may be less often and more difficult. However, these conversations are crucial to the success and well being of your child. There are different approaches that can be taken depending on how you relate to each other, but emphasis on their future is key. Discuss with your child what long term consequences of drug and alcohol abuse look like when they are considering college, or pursuing their future, and the devastating effects that this can have on their life.[5,6]

It's important to provide your teen with a sense of belonging, a respect for commitment and a strong work ethic. Encourage and enable your child to join a sports, gymnastics or martial arts program to create a healthy outlet for frustration, stress and anxiety. Choose family activities that are fun and form a sense of community involvement.[7] Volunteering at a facility that demonstrates the impact of drug use can also provide a visual to the stories, education and information about drugs and abuse.

In my years of clinical practice, I have had numerous students rotate through and many of these students experienced firsthand the problems caused by alcohol and drugs in trauma victims and those with disabling spinal conditions. That experience changed their perspective and significantly shaped their own journey. It is important to consistently praise and affirm your child for the positive choices that are made. **Show genuine interest in their lives** even when the task seems difficult. As a parent, I have found the pursuit of personal happiness is less important than exhibiting behaviors aimed at making the child a better person. Leading by example and practicing selflessness goes a long way in developing positive behaviors in your child.

Discussing drugs, alcohol and sex can be uncomfortable conversations, as well as talking about underage drinking, smoking or dipping tobacco. You may not always know how to approach it or where the conversation will lead. If you begin by finding a relaxed setting alone, you can start with general questions about their interests. There may be resistance in the beginning, especially if they suspect you are going to ask more questions. However, make it a point to listen with empathy and without judgment.

Instead of asking general questions such as: "How was your day, or how was school?" try being more specific with your conversation. Some examples are: "Tell me more about your football practice yesterday" or "Could I see some of your drawings you've been working on lately?" This approach allows your child to feel safe and shows that you are genuinely interested in her activities. Teenagers tend to be very private and secluded at times, so the idea is to give them space **while maintaining an open and safe place for communication**. If by chance, you suspect or they admit to using tobacco, drugs or alcohol, be prepared to speak with them about it.[8]

Make your response as supportive and loving as possible and decide on consequences after you have heard the entire story. If you lose your temper, you may say things you regret, or miss part of the truth of what happened. You will also close the door for future conversations and expend a serious amount of energy trying to find the truth. Various guidance counselors, therapists and drug prevention and treatment websites can assist you in how to deal with specific scenarios. Don't be afraid to reach out for support. Be prepared for anything because teenage life can be a challenge.

XII. Ways to Thrive

"Everything you were looking for was right there with you all the time." **The Wizard of Oz**[1]

There are no guarantees that even if you do all the right things and take all the right steps there won't be problems with your teen. However, it is a worthwhile undertaking as a parent to prepare for that phase of life with your best intention and information. Awareness that leads to positive parental actions does not happen by accident, it takes effort.

Below are eleven suggestions[2] that you can incorporate into your own style of parenting that may help circumvent the possibility of your child becoming another statistic. These suggestions are merely that. A parent's hope is always that their teenager will thrive as an adult. While these strategies are meant to bring awareness and change, it is ultimately up to you. I encourage you to do your part by learning what you can do to help win the battle for your teen.

Following these suggestions, I have additional information composed by a teen about teens that I believe you will find to be open, honest, and real.

1. Lead by Example

Kids are smart. They are a lot more perceptive than they let on. Language is learned by one on one engagement and behaviors are similar. There are many ways that you communicate with your child and he picks up on every one of them. Verbal communication with your children is important and essential, but **they are watching every move you make.** Your actions and demeanors are probably more important than what you say, although kind words backed up by compassion are powerful tools. Every parent lives by a set of rules and behaviors and inevitably passes those principles on to their children.

Children are observant and they will likely adopt the principles they hear and see. Set the example in your own home. If you have a substance abuse problem, take steps to get help and get clean. If by chance you relapse, continue to move forward, forgive yourself and seek help. The effort you put forth to overcome your own personal issues will not only benefit you, but also your family as they see you prevail.

2. Have an Open Line of Communication with Your Children

Keep it safe for your children to have open interaction with you every day even if you don't agree with their perspectives. **This interaction can go a long way in letting them know that you love them, respect their views and want to hear about the details of their day**.

While your kids, especially teenagers, may not share with you uncomfortable or embarrassing topics, let them know they can. Be fair and be real. It is important to have family time, and knowing that their opinion matters will create an atmosphere of harmony and build a level of respect.

Kids need to learn how to communicate without constantly checking the phone for alerts. Help them to develop this necessary skill by enforcing politely, but clearly, that they turn off electronics during conversations. Make it a point to have one-on-one talks on the way to or from school, practice or during family time.

3. Encourage Your Child to Excel at School

Academic excellence comes from hard work, discipline, perseverance and dedication. Generally, kids who exhibit these behaviors and habits lead successful lives as adults and avoid drug addictive behaviors and habits, but it's not a guarantee.

On the other hand, kids who struggle with an unstable family life, lack of parental involvement, academic problems, and other issues all too easily find solace experimenting with drugs and alcohol. Encourage your children to study and read and take school seriously. Start young by reading to your children or letting them read to you every day. Get involved in their academic life. Sacrifice the time and energy necessary to show them that school is important. **Do what is necessary to provide an environment that enables academic success** and maximizes the opportunities for success in the future.

4. Set Guidelines for all Social Media

Parents need to understand that youth today place much of their identity on social media. It has become the social fabric of communication for our youth. **Be cautious and thoughtful about limiting and setting the guidelines for Facebook, Instagram, Snapchat and the myriad of other social media platforms.**

The paradigm of communication has changed with social media activity and though it was revolutionary when you could type a text message and send it without talking, smart phones have replaced the once personal intimate conversations we used to have with one another.

It is essential to have parental control and set boundaries over all of the electronics and the internet-based communication platforms that teens have access to, but be respectful, this is their social identity. Be especially vigilant about their social media behaviors, or other types of on-line communication with virtual relationships.

5. Friend the Friends

Get to know the friends your child is spending time with, their names and the names of their parents. Just as your child's actions and behaviors are a reflection of your own, her friends will also influence her behaviors and habits.

Situational awareness is a requisite for military combat service, and it is also necessary to understand how your child is feeling and what your child is doing. **Be aware of and understand the other potential influences in your child's life.**

6. Do Not Store Pain Pills or Illicit Substances in Your Home

If your doctor prescribes pain pills for a legitimate medical condition, use them as directed and dispose of them when the condition has passed. While it is impossible to shelter your children from all potentially negative influences, it is possible to **make sure your home is not part of the problem.**

Keep prescription pain pills and other controlled substances locked up or inaccessible to your children. Destroy pills that are no longer in active use. You can also take the pills to the pharmacist for safe disposal.

Addicted parents: It is not too late to change course and straighten out your life and the life of your family by seeking treatment. Reading this book is not enough support. If you are a parent and use illicit drugs or drink excessively, protect your children from your inappropriate behaviors by seeking professional help. There are plenty of rehabilitative treatment programs available, and Alcoholics Anonymous is one of many. Break down the disengagement built up by months or years of addiction and ask a friend or family for help. Once children of addicted parents grow into adulthood, the child-parent bonds are often permanently destroyed.

Parents not addicted to substances: diligently protect yourself from alcohol or pain pill dependence. Monitor your own behavior as objectively as possible.

7. Stay Involved and Connected

Do not hesitate to be a parent who volunteers at school, on sports teams or assisting in the classroom. **Show your children that you have an interest in what they are doing** at school or whatever activity or passion they have for the day, week or month.

If you are too busy or just not interested, your child will perceive that lack of interest and may look elsewhere for that bond. Being too busy, whether it's work duties or otherwise, does not compare to the personal time and interest that you can invest in your child.

8. Encourage Your Child to Stay Active

Anxiety and stress, if left unattended, can develop into a more serious problem. Each person is affected differently. Enrolling your child into an activity program may allow him to excel, help alleviate stress and may become therapeutic. Positive activities that go beyond school work, video games or just hanging out with friends can serve as outlets and will likely deter boredom and idle down time. Let your children choose the activity to participate in and they will likely stay with it. **If they choose it, they will own it**.

Dance, sports, arts and crafts, music, fishing and hiking are all positive activities that create a healthy outlet for your child to properly channel frustration and anxiety.

9. Get on Board with Volunteering

Have your child connect with a volunteer program that enables him to participate and envision a bigger purpose in life. The benefit of volunteering will provide confidence, security, purpose and ultimately replace the feelings of self-doubt, self-hatred and self-defeat.

We live in a world where many kids believe they are entitled, which creates a more negative mindset in teens. **Volunteering will help your children learn love, and develop empathy and acceptance of others as well as themselves.**

If volunteering is not possible or practical, then helping your teen find a job that helps others is a good substitute.

10. Don't Be Afraid to Talk about Drug Use

Talking about unanticipated consequences of life choices can be uncomfortable at best, but always better discussed beforehand. The same goes with the consequences that occur from casual drug use.

Become educated about drug abuse and its consequences in your community and stay knowledgeable about the current trends. The increasing availability of the super-potent and deadly Fentanyl is the wakeup call for every parent. **Make sure your children understand that the dangers of drug abuse are real** and be prepared to state your case with facts that are readily available from a variety of sources including your own neighborhood. Don't be afraid of the discussion. Chances are your child has more than a passing knowledge about the reality of drug abuse.

11. Be the Parent

Friends are important and necessary for sound social development. While you may have a great friendship with your child, it's important to know that these circumstances require you to be a respected and authoritative parent. **Kids thrive on parental guidance with set boundaries**.

As a parent, you are a teacher, counselor, caretaker and coach who must be willing to go the distance and against the grain to correct them when necessary. This means they won't always like you. They won't always care for what you say, and they won't always agree with your decisions. That's okay. **Being a loving and affirming parent means more than universally accepting your child's actions and decisions.**

Develop guidelines and boundaries of acceptable behaviors and actions. Be prepared to affirm with love when the rules are followed, and be prepared to correct with love when boundaries have been broken.

While there is no perfect solution and no guarantees, these suggestions and methods have a higher success rate with keeping teens off drugs and helping them build a solid foundation to live a healthy, happy and productive life. Training your child to live with intention, purpose and accountability will render greater joy in your family, community and society.

◆ ◆ ◆

It's one thing for a person in my position, as a parent, physician and surgeon, to offer a guide with suggestions that will hopefully steer your child away from the life-changing consequences of drug or alcohol abuse, but to fully comprehend the nuances of this issue, it's necessary to understand those we are trying to reach.

Realistically, our teenager's world is not our world. We may have walked a similar road and hopefully gained wisdom with our experience, but each generation encounters unique challenges that must be navigated. The world of today's youth looks very little like the world we knew when we were young.

◆ ◆ ◆

As a final bonus, I have included a teen's perspective on how to have a healthy relationship with your teen and the support that will help get them through these vulnerable years and the pressures that they encounter.

A Teen's Perspective
By Natalie Sanders

1. Establish a working relationship with your kid.

Sounds easy, right? Well, don't be surprised when your teenager would prefer to go out with friends or, more commonly, spend time in their rooms, locked up with a book or TV show. Look, we're still figuring this whole "life" stuff out (and so are you, if you feel you need to read a guide about how to keep your kids off drugs).

School isn't just physically tiring—it latches onto your brain and drains you emotionally. Some days, the thought of any more human interaction after school makes us go our own kind of insane. This will not - I repeat, will not - be cured by any sort of questioning about how our day went.

Trust me, if something awesome happened at school, we would tell you. Instead, try to ease your way into a conversation by talking about things other than academics, or if your kid has a crush on that girl/boy, or why they look so tired. Talk about that awesome movie that people can't shut up about. Or how your co-worker laughed so hard she had to lay down and count to ten. Or something casual. Try different starters, and see what works. Any verbal response is a mission success.

Teenagers are not going to be real with you if you are not real with them, so my advice is not to treat them like they hardly know anything, or their issues aren't important.

While still being a parental figure, look at any situation from all angles and try to put yourself in our position. Once you can have a casual conversation, then round back to things like school or relationships. Keep it real. Establish some wiggle room between the layers of heartfelt-sarcasm and teenage-angst that makes up your child sitting quietly in the passenger seat. Put your flag in it, like the astronauts did. Claim it yours. This is your relationship. This is the start of everything.

2. Anxiety and depression do some crazy damage.

Kids do irresponsible stuff, like drugs or drinking, when they get desperate. It's the gospel truth. So how do you keep your teenager from getting desperate? Good question.

I guess we have to go back to that wiggle room of a relationship you have hopefully managed to establish. No one knows your kid like you do, so start noticing things. Are they eating? Are they sleeping too much or not at all? Are they having problems fitting in? Anxiety issues are common for teenagers, but sometimes it causes very real, very serious problems in everyday life. It can keep us shut off, glued to a textbook, or ignoring school entirely.

Ask us how we are. When we give our vague, ambiguous answer of "fine," ask us again. Make eye contact. Show us that you're genuinely concerned with our mental state. Show us that you recognize our problems are real and see if there's anything you can do to help manage stress or other common problems. Do whatever you can to keep your child mentally and emotionally healthy, whether it be talking it out or just LISTENING. Sometimes we don't want to talk about it. Sadly, not much can be done in this situation except to let them know that you're there for them, and keep fighting for that little pocket of a relationship. It gets better and bigger with time and trust.

3. Be the parent.

Now for the really hard stuff. How are you supposed to know how much freedom is too much? Or how much grace to extend when we mess up (again)? If only there was some scientific formula we could use. I guess you can only start with a few key notes and work your way up from there.

4. Let your kid have opinions.

This is pretty self-explanatory. Teens are figuring out who they are and what they believe in. Let them. Make your own opinions known and explain why you think that way, but don't force them to believe something.

5. Give them resources.

Give your kids resources to succeed in school, social situations, and more. This can come in the form of a book, a person, a job opportunity, or your own personal advice.

6. Guide them.

Step in when the kid is about to do something you know can't end well. Put on your parent face and tell them, firmly, no. Tell them why you said no. Listen to their side of the story. Reiterate. This is your kid. Your kid doesn't have this all figured out. Help them, even if they don't want to be helped.

7. Keep working on your relationship.

Make that little space into a football arena. Fight and make up. Always make up. Try not to have loose-ends. Remember that we're far from perfect, but we are trying. Show us that you are too

Below is a list of references for guidance and support when dealing with possible drug addiction and how to manage its many issues and faces. These support links are materials to initiate counseling to help prevent or manage the disease of addiction, but these resources are not intended to replace seeking a professional family therapist trained in substance abuse.

Support & Help Links:

1. www.drugfree.org
2. www.drugabuse.gov
3. www.getsmartaboutdrugs.gov
4. www.preventteendruguse.org
5. www.addictionsandrecovery.org
6. www.healthychildren.org
7. www.therecoveryvillage.com
8. www.mayoclinic.org
9. www.ncadd.org
10. www.narconon.org

References:

Intro:

1. NPR. "Obama Shares Plans to Tackle Heroin Epidemic in West Virginia." All Things Considered, by Don Gonyea, 21 Oct 2015, http://www.npr.org/2015/10/21/4506117 79/obama-shares-plans-to-tackle-heroin-epidemic-in-west-virginia. 20 Mar 2017.
2. HelpGuide.org. "Understanding Addiction." Harvard Mental Health Letter and Overcoming Addiction: Paths toward recovery, a special health report published by Harvard Health Publications, (Na, nd), https://www.helpguide.org/harvard/how-addiction-hijacks-the-brain.htm. 20 March 2017.
3. The Washington Post. "Congress Passes 21st Century Cures Act, Boosting Research and Easing Drug Approvals." Power Post, by Mike DeBonis, 7 Dec 2016, https://www.washingtonpost.com/news/

powerpost/wp/2016/12/07/congress-passes-21st-century-cures-act-boosting-research-and-easing-drug-approvals/?utm_term=.c49f7c638142. 20 March 2017.

4. ProjectKnow. "How Teens are Exposed to Drugs and Alcohol." For Teens, by Brittany Tackett, MA, (nd), http://www.projectknow.com/research/drugs-and-alcohol/. 22 Mar 2017.

Chapt. I

1. Business Insider. "Here's an Amazing Scene from 'Louie' In Which Joan Rivers Explains Why She's a Comedian." By Aly Weisman. 4 Sept 2014, http://www.businessinsider.com/joan-rivers-explanation-of-why-shes-a-comedian-on-louie-2014-9. 2 Feb 2017.

2. Healthline. "Recognizing an Addiction Problems." Newsletter, by Mara Tyler, 23 June 2016,

http://www.healthline.com/health/addicti
on/recognizing-addiction#early-signs2.
23 Mar 2017.

3. Redeye. "Life as a Recovering Addict."
Chicago Tribune, by Leonor Vivanco. 28
Sept 2015,
http://www.chicagotribune.com/redeye/r
edeye-addiction-national-recovery-
month-september-20150926-story.html.
1 Mar 2017.

Chapt. II

1. Every Quotes. Justin Timberlake about
Teen, (nd),
https://www.everywishes.com/quotes/qu
ote/56068/6135. 4 Feb 2017.
2. CDC. "Mortality among Teenagers Aged
12-19 Years: United States, 1999-2006."
By Arialdi M. Minino, M.P.H., 5 May
2010,
https://www.cdc.gov/nchs/products/data
briefs/db37.html. 6 Feb 2017.
3. CDC. "Excessive Drinking is Draining
the US Economy." Centers for Disease
Control and Prevention, 12 Jan 2016,

https://www.cdc.gov/features/costsofdrinking/index.html. 6 Feb 2017.

4. NIH. "Underage Drinking." National Institute on Alcohol Abuse and Alcoholism, Feb 2017, https://pubs.niaaa.nih.gov/publications/UnderageDrinking/UnderageFact.htm. 2 Mar 2017.

5. NIH. "Underage Drinking." National Institute on Alcohol Abuse and Alcoholism, Feb 2017, https://pubs.niaaa.nih.gov/publications/underagedrinking/Underage_Fact.pdf. 2 March 2017.

6. NPR. "Teen Drinking May Cause Irreversible Brain Damage." National Public Radio, by Michelle Trudeau, January 25, 2010, http://www.npr.org/templates/story/story.php?storyId=122765890. 22 Mar 2017.

7. American Addiction Centers. "Short and Long Term Mental Effects of Alcohol." Alcohol Addiction Treatment, (Na, Nd), http://americanaddictioncenters.org/alcoholism-treatment/mental-effects/. 16 Feb 2017.

8. Trauma Abuse Treatment. "Lowered Inhibitions and Alcohol." Trauma Abuse Treatment, (Na, nd) http://traumaabusetreatment.com/lowered-inhibitions-and-alcohol-abuse. 16 Feb 2017.

9. Drinkaware. "Understand Why Children Drink Alcohol." Underage Drinking, (Na, nd), https://www.drinkaware.co.uk/advice/underage-drinking/understand-why-children-drink-alcohol/. 6 Mar 2017.

10. NIH. "Underage Drinking." National Institute on Alcohol Abuse and Alcoholism, (Na) Feb 2017, https://pubs.niaaa.nih.gov/publications/underagedrinking/Underage_Fact.pdf. 8 Mar 2017.

11. The Right Step. "Is Your Teen Abusing Alcohol or Drugs? What You Can do to Help." Teen Drug Addiction, (Na), 1 July 2014, https://www.rightstep.com/teen-drug-addiction/how-to-help-your-abusing-teen/. 6 Mar 2017.

Chapt. III

1. BBC. "Lao Tzu, Moving Words, (nd). Archived page. http://www.bbc.co.uk/worldservice/learningenglish/movingwords/shortlist/laotzu.shtml. 3 Mar 2017.
2. HuffPost. "16 Wildly Successful People Who Overcame Huge Obstacles to Get There." Healthy Living, by Renee Jacques, 8 Nov 2016, http://www.huffingtonpost.com/2013/09/25/successful-people-obstacles_n_3964459.html. 8 Mar 2017.
3. Learning Lift Off. "Overcoming Obstacles: How FDR's Paralysis Made Him a Better President." Lifestyles, Live & Learn, by Elizabeth Street, 15, Jan 2015, http://www.learningliftoff.com/overcoming-obstacles-how-fdrs-paralysis-made-him-a-better-president/#.WUglimjyvIU. 10 Mar 2017.
4. NBA. "My Amazing Journey: LeBron James." NBA.Com 2007-2008, (Na, nd), http://www.nba.com/preview2007/journey_james.html. 10 Mar 2017.
5. Encyclopedia of World Biography. "Oprah Winfrey Biography." World

Biography, (nd),
http://www.notablebiographies.com/We-Z/Winfrey-Oprah.html. 8 Mar 2017.

6. Parents. "Failure is an Option." Parents Magazine, by Aviva Patz, (nd), http://www.parents.com/kids/development/behavioral/failure-is-an-option/. 2 Mar 2017.

Chapt. IV

1. Lakers Nation. "Top Five Kobe Bryant Quotes." News, by Steve Almazan, 16 June 2011, http://www.lakersnation.com/top-five-kobe-bryant-quotes/2011/06/16/2/. 3 Mar 2017.

2. CBS News. "Teen Drug Abuse: 14 Mistakes Parents Make." CBS News, by Dr. Joseph Lee, (nd), http://www.cbsnews.com/pictures/teen-drug-abuse-14-mistakes-parents-make/. 30 Jan 2017.

3. Very Well. "Tough Love in Parenting Troubled Teens." Teens, by Kathryn Rudlin, LCSW, 31, Jan 2017, https://www.verywell.com/tough-love-in-

parenting-troubled-teens-2610430. 4 Jan 2017.

4. Family Matters Parenting Magazine. "Tough Love Parenting: When & How to Use Tough Love Parenting." Parenting Child Development, (Na, nd), http://www.parenting-child-development.com/tough-love-parenting.html. 30 Jan 2017.

5. Help Your Teen Now. "Tough Love Strategies in Parenting Troubled Teens." Help Your Teen Now, 27 Jan 2016, http://helpyourteennow.com/tough-love-strategies-in-parenting-troubled-teens/. 28 Jan 2017.

6. WAHM.Com. "5 Tips to Reach Out to Your Rebellious Teen." Wahm articles, Work-at-home-moms, (nd), http://www.wahm.com/articles/5-tips-to-reach-out-to-your-rebellious-teen.html. 22 Jan 2017.

Chapt. V

1. The Washington Post. "Nelson Mandela on the Power of Education." Answer

Sheet, by Valerie Strauss, 5 Dec 2013, https://www.washingtonpost.com/news/answer-sheet/wp/2013/12/05/nelson-mandelas-famous-quote-on-education/?utm_term=.8ccc4c7c20d7. 23 Jan 2017.

2. DrugrehabUS. "Prescription Drugs Claim More Lives Than Illegal Street Drugs." Elements Behavioral Health, (Na, nd), http://www.drugrehab.us/news/prescription-drugs-street-drugs/. 28 Jan 2017.

3. NIDA. "Research on the Use and Misuse of Fentanyl and Other Synthetic Opioids." National Institute on Drug Abuse, presented by Wilson M. Compton, M.D., 21 Mar 2017, https://www.drugabuse.gov/about-nida/legislative-activities/testimony-to-congress/2017/research-use-misuse-fentanyl-other-synthetic-opioids. 28 Mar 2017.

4. WSB-TV Atlanta."Urgent Warning Issued About Deadly Counterfeit Drug." Channel 2 Action News, by Tom Regan, 10 Mar 2016, http://www.wsbtv.com/news/2-

investigates/urgent-warning-issued-about-deadly-counterfeit-drug/149537903. 30 Mar 2017.

5. The Recovery Village. "Xanax Addiction." Recovery Blog, (Na, nd), https://www.therecoveryvillage.com/xanax-addiction/. 28 Feb 2017.

6. NIDA. "Opioids are driving increase in cocaine overdose deaths." National Institute on Drug Abuse, 9 Feb. 2017, https://www.drugabuse.gov/news-events/news-releases/2017/02/opioids-are-driving-increase-in-cocaine-overdose-deaths. 2 Mar 2017.

7. NIDA. "Prescription Opioids and Heroin." National Institute on Drug Abuse, 16 Dec. 2015, https://www.drugabuse.gov/publications/research-reports/prescription-opioids-heroin.
2 Mar 2017.

8. Mayo Clinic. "Prescription Drug Abuse." Diseases and Conditions, by Mayo Clinic Staff, 19 Sept 2015, http://www.mayoclinic.org/diseases-conditions/prescription-drug-

abuse/basics/definition/con-20032471.
26 Feb 2017.

9. Very Well. "Using Drugs Without a
   Prescription is Illegal." Prescription
   Medication, by Buddy T., 23 April 2017,
   https://www.verywell.com/using-drugs-
   without-a-prescription-is-illegal-69457. 6
   June 2017.

Chapt. VI

1. "drug of choice." Dictionary.com's 21st
   Century Lexicon. Dictionary.com, LLC
   23 June 2017. <Dictionary.com,
   http://www.dictionary.com/browse/drug-
   of-choice>
2. Foundation for a Drug-Free World.
   "Painkillers: A Short History." The Truth
   About Painkillers, (Na, nd),
   http://www.drugfreeworld.org/drugfacts/
   painkillers/a-short-history.html. 16 Jan
   2017.
3. CDC. "Prescription Opioids." Opioid
   Basics, (Na), 16 Mar 2016,
   https://www.cdc.gov/drugoverdose/opioi
   ds/prescribed.html. 6 Feb 2017.

4. Opium. " What Are Synthetic Opioids."
   Opium.org, (Na, nd),
   http://www.opium.org/what-are-
   synthetic-opioids.html. 28 Jan 2017.
5. CNN. "Death from Synthetic Opioids up
   72%, CDC says." Health: Parenting &
   Family, by Debra Goldschmidt, 16 Dec
   2016,
   http://www.cnn.com/2016/12/16/health/s
   ynthetic-opioid-deaths/. 26 Jan 2017.
6. Foundation for a Drug-Free World. "The
   Truth About Prescription Drug
   Abuse/International Statistics." Drug
   Free World, (Na, nd),
   http://www.drugfreeworld.org/drugfacts/
   prescription/abuse-international-
   statistics.html. 20 Feb 2017.
7. CDC. "Understanding the Epidemic."
   Centers for Disease Control and
   Prevention, Opioid Overdose, 16 Dec
   2016,
   https://www.cdc.gov/drugoverdose/epid
   emic/. 4 Feb 2017.
8. Addictionblog.org."The Six Most
   Dangerous Synthetic Drugs."Drug, by
   Warren Rivera, 3 Aug 2016,
   http://drug.addictionblog.org/the-6-most-

dangerous-synthetic-drugs-on-the-market/. 20 Jan 2017.

9. Rxlist. "Narcan." Rxlist, Narcan Side Effects Center, medical editor, John P. Cunha, DO, FACOEP, 16 Sept 2016, http://www.rxlist.com/narcan-side-effects-drug-center.htm. 6 June 2017.

10. Foundation for a Drug-Free World. "The Truth about Synthetic Drugs." Drug Free World, (Na, nd), http://www.drugfreeworld.org/drugfacts/synthetic.html. 8 Jan 2017.

11. Live Science. "What is THC?." Health, by Alina Bradfort, Live Science Contributor, 18 May 2017, http://www.livescience.com/24553-what-is-thc.html. 13 Jan 2017.

12. NIDA. "Synthetic Cannabinoids." National Institute on Drug Abuse, 9 Nov. 2015, https://www.drugabuse.gov/publications/drugfacts/synthetic-cannabinoids. 15 Jan 2017.

13. CADCA. "Synthetic Drugs." Community Anti-Drug Coalitions of America, (Na, nd), http://www.cadca.org/synthetic-drugs. 13 Feb 2017.

14. Business Insider. "A Handful of Dangerous New Legal Drugs has Public Health Experts Worried." Science, by Matthew Speiser, 11 Aug 2015, http://www.businessinsider.com/new-synthetic-drugs-2015-8. 18 Feb 2017.
15. Rolling Stone. "Florida Zombie Drug Flakka: Everything You Need to Know." News, by Annamarya Scaccia, 19 Aug 2016, http://www.rollingstone.com/culture/news/florida-zombie-drug-flakka-everything-you-need-to-know-w435074. 22 Feb 2017.
16. Broward.org."Flakka Frequently Asked Questions."Broward Addiction Recovery, (Na, nd), http://www.broward.org/HumanServices/BrowardAddictionRecovery/Pages/FlakkaFAQ.aspx. 22 Feb 2017.
17. MedicineNet.com. "Flakka." Mental Health, medical author, John P. Cunha, DO, FACOEP, medical editor, Charles Patrick Davis, M.D., PhD., 1 Dec 2016, http://www.medicinenet.com/flakka/article.htm;

http://www.medicinenet.com/flakka/page 2.htm. 23 Feb 2017.

Chapt. VII

1. DrugAbuse.com. "Shocking Stories Reveal Serious Dangers of Flakka." Drugabuse.com, (Na, nd), http://drugabuse.com/shocking-stories-reveal-serious-dangers-of-flakka/. 21 Feb 2017.
2. Broward.org. "Flakka Frequently Asked Questions." Broward Addiction Recovery, (Na, nd), http://www.broward.org/HumanServices/BrowardAddictionRecovery/Pages/FlakkaFAQ.aspx. 25 Feb 2017.
3. CNN. "Progress Against Chinese Chemists Selling Dangerous Synthetic Drugs in US." Health: Parenting & Family, by Sara Ganim, CNN, 2 Sept 2016, http://www.cnn.com/2016/09/02/health/chinese-selling-synthetic-drugs-in-us-down/. 23 Feb 2017.

4. http://www.cnn.com/2016/09/02/health/chinese-selling-synthetic-drugs-in-us-down/

5. NIDA. "Fentanyl." National Institute on Drug Abuse, (Na) 6 Jun. 2016, https://www.drugabuse.gov/drugs-abuse/fentanyl. 28 Mar 2017.

6. DrugAbuse.com. "Snorting Fentanyl." Library, by Eric Patterson, MSCP, NCC, LPC, (nd), http://drugabuse.com/library/snorting-fentanyl/. 26 Mar 2017.

7. Foundation for a Drug-Free World. "What is LSD?." Drug-Free World, The Truth About LSD, (Na, nd), http://www.drugfreeworld.org/drugfacts/lsd.html. 4 Mar 2017.

8. NIDA. "MDMA (Ecstasy/Molly)." National Institute on Drug Abuse, (Na) 12 Oct. 2016, https://www.drugabuse.gov/publications/drugfacts/mdma-ecstasymolly. 3 Mar 2017.

Chapt. VIII

1. Partnership for Drug-Free Kids. "Talk With Your Kids." Medicine Abuse Project, (Na, nd), https://drugfree.org/article/talk-with-your-kids/. 7 Feb 2017.

2. Narconon. "How to Talk to Your Kids About Drugs." Parent Center, (Na, nd), http://www.narconon.org/drug-abuse/talking-to-kids-about-drugs.html. 5 Feb 2017.

3. NIDA. "Principles of Adolescent Substance Use Disorder Treatment: A Research-Based Guide." National Institute on Drug Abuse, (Na) 14 Jan. 2014, https://www.drugabuse.gov/publications/principles-adolescent-substance-use-disorder-treatment-research-based-guide. 14 Jan 2017.

4. AddictionCenter. "Statistics of Addiction in America."Addiction Statistics, (Na, nd), https://www.addictioncenter.com/addiction/addiction-statistics/. 29 Jan 2017.

5. The Recovery Village. "How to Talk to Your Kids About Drugs." The Friends and Family Portal, (Na, nd),

https://www.therecoveryvillage.com/family-friend-portal/talking-about-drugs/#gref. 2 Feb 2017.

Chapt. IX

1. Mumford & Sons. "The Cave." By Marcus Oliver Johnstone Mumford, Edward James Milton Dwane, Benjamin Walter David Lovett and Winston Aubrey Aladar Marshall. *Sigh No More.*
2. Narconon. "The Five Most Common Traits of an Addict." Drug Abuse Info, (Na, nd), http://www.narconon.org/blog/drug-addiction/5-common-behavior-traits-addict/ and http://www.narconon.org/drug-abuse/signs-symptoms-of-drug-abuse.html. 21 Feb 2017.
3. New York State and the Office of Alcoholism and Substance Abuse Service. "How to Know: I think my child is using alcohol and/or drugs." (Na, nd), https://www.health.ny.gov/publications/1089.pdf. 22 Feb 2017.

4. Drug Abuse.Com. "Symptoms and Signs of Drug Abuse." Reviewed by Joe Houchins, M.A., http://drugabuse.com/library/symptoms-and-signs-of-drug-abuse/. 21 Feb 2017.

Chapt. X

1. Esquire. "What I've Learned: Eric Clapton." By Cal Fussman, 6 Oct 2014, http://www.esquire.com/entertainment/music/interviews/a4017/eric-clapton0108/.
2. NCADD. "Signs and Symptoms." National Council on Alcoholism and Drug Dependence, 19 Dec 2016, https://www.ncadd.org/about-addiction/signs-and-symptoms/signs-and-symptoms. 10 Feb 2017.
3. NCADD. "Signs and Symptoms." National Council on Alcoholism and Drug Dependence, 19 Dec 2016, https://www.ncadd.org/about-addiction/signs-and-symptoms/signs-and-symptoms. 10 Feb 2017.
4. NIDA. "What to do if Your Teen or Young Adult Has a Problem With Drugs." National Institute on Drug

Abuse, Revised Jan. 2016,
https://www.drugabuse.gov/related-
topics/treatment/what-to-do-if-your-teen-
or-young-adult-has-problem-drugs. 15
Feb 2017.

Chapt. XI

1. NIDA. "Principles of Adolescent
   Substance Use Disorder Treatment: A
   Research-Based Guide." National
   Institute on Drug Abuse, (Na) 14 Jan.
   2014,
   https://www.drugabuse.gov/publications/
   principles-adolescent-substance-use-
   disorder-treatment-research-based-
   guide. 21 Jan 2017.
2. NPR. "Today's Heroin Addict is Young,
   White And Surburban." Shots Health
   News from NPR (National Public Radio),
   by Maanvi Singh, 28 May 2014,
   http://www.npr.org/sections/health-
   shots/2014/05/28/316673753/todays-
   heroin-addict-is-young-white-and-
   suburban. 8 Jan 2017.
3. The Recovery Village. "Drug Use in
   High School." Teen Addiction, (Na, nd),

https://www.therecoveryvillage.com/teen-addiction/how-do-teens-get-drugs/#gref. 10 Jan 2017.

4. Partnership for Drug-Free Kids. "What to Say to Your Teenager about Drugs." Prevention Tips for Every Age, (Na, nd), https://drugfree.org/article/prevention-tips-for-every-age/#tips4. 8 Jan 2017.

5. DrugAbuse.com. "Drug Abuse Prevention." Prevention, (Na, nd), http://drugabuse.com/library/drug-abuse-prevention/. 8 Jan 2017.

6. Partnership for Drug-Free Kids. "Prevention Tips for Every Age." http://www.drugfree.org/the-parent-toolkit/age-by-age-advice/16-18-year-old-what-to-say/. 21 Feb 2017.

7. The Atlantic. "How Iceland got Teens to Say No to Drugs." Health, by Emma Young, 19 Jan 2017, https://www.theatlantic.com/health/archive/2017/01/teens-drugs-iceland/513668/. 2 Mar 2017.

8. Phoenix House. "Simple Methods to Prevent Your Teen from Using Drugs or Alcohol." New & Events, (Na) 19 Sept 2012,

https://www.phoenixhouse.org/news-and-views/news-and-events/simple-methods-to-prevent-your-teen-from-using-drugs-or-alcohol/. 23 Feb 2017

Chapt. XII

1. "The Wizard of Oz." Dir Victor Fleming, George Cukor. Metro-Goldwyn-Mayer, 1939. Film.
2. Mayo Clinic. "Teen Drug Abuse: Help Your Teen Avoid Drugs." By Mayo Clinic Staff, 2 Feb. 2016, http://www.mayoclinic.org/healthy-lifestyle/tween-and-teen-health/in-depth/teen-drug -abuse/art-20045921. 21 Jan 2017.

64643789R00060

Made in the USA
Middletown, DE
16 February 2018